DISCOVER GOD'S HEALTH WISDOM

DISCOVER GOD'S HEALTH WISDOM

Exposing 8 Common Myths That Keep You Sick

ALEXANDRA YU

Contents

Who Has the Right Answers for My Health? 11

Part 1: Eight Health Myths That Keep You Sick

1. If a Health Protocol Worked for Someone Else,
It Will Work for Me Too 17

2. If the Treatment Didn't Harm Someone Else,
It Won't Harm Me Either 21

3. If the Drug Stopped the Symptom, My Health
Has Improved 27

4. If I Want to Eliminate My Health Symptoms, I Only
Need to Focus on the Physical Needs of My Body 31

5. Natural Treatments and Nonconventional Methods
Do Not Work 45

6. My Body Is Inherently Dysfunctional, and There's
Nothing Anyone Can Do About It 51

7. I Can Sit Back and Let the Medical System Take Care of Me . . 57

8. The Bible Has Nothing to Say about My Health 67

Part 2: How Can We Experience True Healing?

9. Have Faith and Ask God for Wisdom 75

10. Know the Truth and Meditate on the Truth 87

11. Pray for a Change of Heart, Ears to Hear, and Eyes to See . . 95

12. Be Obedient and Trust God with the Outcome 103

Who Has the Right Answers for My Health?

*"Call to me and I will answer you, and will tell you
great and hidden things that you have not known."*

JEREMIAH 33:3

"Wow, your legs are like sticks!" This was a refrain I heard often in my youth. I've always been on the thin side. Growing up, adults would tell me, "I used to look like you. You might as well eat whatever you want now because when you get older, you won't be thin anymore." I took their advice and basically ate whatever I wanted. I hated vegetables, and only ate them because my mom cooked them and coaxed me into eating them each day.

In high school, I was on the track team, and I started working out to sculpt my body—more for vanity than for health reasons. Other than my relationship with God, working out, and my mom's attempts to persuade me to eat healthy foods, my other routines were not healthy. I was a moody kid who came home and fell asleep in front of the

TV. I was often fatigued because I was a chronic procrastinator who stayed up late every night to maintain good grades.

In college, my diet consisted of processed foods and artificial sweeteners. I ate anything that was cheap, microwavable, or convenient. I was still thin with no visible health problems. (Although, looking back, I now know that my diet definitely affected my well-being, especially my emotional health.) In nursing school, a friend who loved healthy foods told me that she always saw me eating food out of a package. I remember thinking, *What else is there to eat? It's easy to grab a Pop-Tart and run out the door. I don't know what else to pack.*

When I started working in the pharmaceutical industry, I would eat four frozen, salty, highly processed microwavable burgers for lunch in one sitting. I thought, *Hey, I'm still thin. I can eat whatever I want and be healthy.*

When I was older and started to have recurring health issues, I changed my diet and was delighted to learn that God's healthy foods and natural remedies—God's provision for his people—were effective at healing the body. As I continued working as a nurse in the clinical research industry, I became reluctantly aware that our culture's views about food, health treatments, and the body are often not formulated by the wisest principles. This realization may lead someone to ask, "Who can I trust when it comes to my health?" or "Who has the right answers for my health?"

About a year ago, someone asked me what I love about nursing. At first, I told her that I didn't love nursing. Unfortunately, sometimes my lofty dream of helping people feels crushed underneath a crap-load of unhelpful medical dogma, bureaucracy, censorship, and corruption. That's the worn out, jaded, "good people don't win in this world" side of me talking. But as I reflected on her question, the other side of me—the wide-eyed, hopeful, "Jesus has already won the battle" side—realized that there are at least two things that I appreciate about nursing: (1) I value how nursing can provide a glimpse into what is really important in life, and (2) I love the privilege of being an advocate for my patients.

You are not my patient, but you picked up this book for a reason. Is it possible that you need extra support with your health? For now, pretend that I am your nurse—your advocate. As your advocate, I invite you to examine your beliefs about your body and your health. Where do your beliefs come from? Do they align with your values? Do they align with the Bible?

True, lasting change often starts with a mindset shift. This book will challenge you to examine your views on health so that you can experience the freedom that God intended for you long before you were even born. This book will ultimately encourage you to seek wisdom and wholeness from the one who created you—the most powerful, loving healer.

PART 1

EIGHT HEALTH MYTHS THAT KEEP YOU SICK

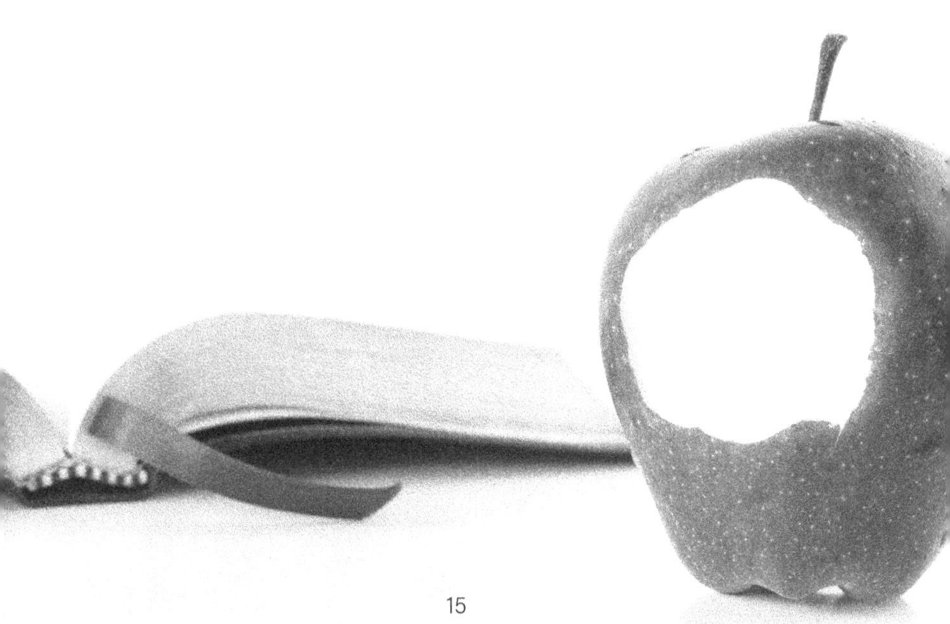

If a Health Protocol Worked for Someone Else, It Will Work for Me Too

"For you formed my inward parts; you knitted me together in my mother's womb. I praise you, for I am fearfully and wonderfully made. Wonderful are your works; my soul knows it very well. My frame was not hidden from you, when I was being made in secret, intricately woven in the depths of the earth. Your eyes saw my unformed substance; in your book were written, every one of them, the days that were formed for me, when as yet there was none of them."

PSALM 139:13-16

During a company presentation, a medical doctor compared his job as a physician to the task of a worker on an assembly line. Doctors are often forced to quickly diagnose and treat patients using algorithms and protocols created by health authorities. This approach may be effective for robots, but it is ineffective—and often dangerous—for humans. God made each one of us unique, and we all live in diverse environments.

For example, many people rave about a particular diet. One person says that he lost one hundred pounds on a vegan diet, another reveals that she finally became pregnant after starting the paleo diet, and another person shares that his cancer vanished after switching to a ketogenic diet.

Just because a specific diet, herb, or supplement benefits some people does not mean that it will be helpful for everyone. My new health-care practitioner told me that she switched to a vegan diet for a year, and it was the worst year of health she had ever experienced. Some people believe the paleo diet does not include important food groups that all people need. A woman I know tried the ketogenic diet for a while, but she noticed more health benefits when she switched to a plant-based diet.

It is also worth noting that since one's health depends on multiple factors, a health protocol that works as a "magic bullet" once may not work the next time. Our unique circumstances, emotional states, and physical needs are always changing. Therefore, if we want vibrant health, the wisest thing to do *first* is ask God for wisdom on the best way to move forward with our health.

In addition to praying, it is also wise to become students of our own bodies. I like to say, "Be your own lab rat." For example, when I had an itchy, painful skin flare (rashes on my face, neck, underarms, arms, hands, and foot), an essential oil cleanse helped my skin immensely. Months later, when I had another flare, the rashes went away after I started consuming more bone broth and coconut oil. A few months after that, when my skin broke out again following a prolonged period of stress, I increased my intake of raw dairy and fermented foods, and the rashes disappeared within one week.

Sometimes we find what our bodies need through trial and error. And because the needs of our bodies change, we may have to make adjustments—what worked in one season may not work in the next season. Medical testing prescribed by a healthcare professional can also be helpful, but we need to remember that these tests are not always accurate. Medical tests are data points that can be misinterpreted or misunderstood. That is why I want to emphasize this point again: we must ask God for wisdom when it comes to our health. As James 1:5–8 advises us:

> If any of you lacks wisdom, let him ask God, who gives generously to all without reproach, and it will be given him. But let him ask in faith, with no doubting, for the one who doubts is like a wave of the sea that is driven and tossed by the wind. For that person must not suppose that he will receive anything from the Lord; he is a double-minded man, unstable in all his ways.

If the Treatment Didn't Harm Someone Else, It Won't Harm Me Either

"Be sober-minded; be watchful. Your adversary the devil prowls around like a roaring lion, seeking someone to devour. Resist him, firm in your faith, knowing that the same kinds of suffering are being experienced by your brotherhood throughout the world. And after you have suffered a little while, the God of all grace, who has called you to his eternal glory in Christ, will himself restore, confirm, strengthen, and establish you. To him be the dominion forever and ever. Amen."

1 PETER 5:8-11

Evangeline knows how it feels to experience extreme harm from medical treatment. She shared her experience after receiving a preventive treatment, "Within a month, my hair started falling out. I was hungry all the time. I was always sharp academically, but now I had horrible brain fog. I couldn't put two and two together. My nursing professor asked me a question and I didn't even know what she was saying. That's how bad it was. It just got so bad that I had to drop out of nursing school."

One day, my dad and I were talking about the medical field, which led to a discussion about pharmaceutical ads on TV. He said, "They always display soothing music with patients dancing around in meadows. But they don't even have enough time in the commercial to get through the never-ending list of side effects." In the United States, we have largely become desensitized to the fact that pharmaceuticals can have enormous negative consequences—like they did for Evangeline who had to drop out of nursing school. How much do we really know about the treatments we put into our bodies each day? And if we experience symptoms, do we stop to consider whether our symptoms are actually caused by something that our doctors prescribed to us? Are medical teams properly trained on the adverse events listed on the drug labels? Unfortunately, my friend who had to leave nursing school experienced severe side effects after receiving a standard, routine treatment that is prescribed to countless numbers of people.

God made the body amazingly complex, and I believe that mere humans—including those in the medical field—understand only a fraction of all there is to know about it. We are such ignorant creatures in comparison to God. Therefore, if a healthcare provider tells us with certainty, "Your new symptom is in no way related to this new treatment," should we be so quick to believe them? Most healthcare providers may have good intentions, but unfortunately, not much of what they say is based upon wisdom from God. Rather, their professional opinions may be based upon clever marketing, opinions from like-minded experts, or biased scientific research that has potentially been manipulated for financial gain.

Before I started working in clinical research, I was under the impression that clinical studies were performed with the utmost integrity. Unfortunately, from years of firsthand experience in this industry, I have seen high turnover rates, a severe lack of communication, apathy, dishonesty, and a lack of accountability. You would think that when companies receive a slap on the wrist for cutting corners or for missing regulatory deadlines, they would learn to be more responsible and vigilant. I have seen the opposite happen—they look for loopholes so that they can put in the least amount of time, money, and effort to "fix" what needed fixing.

You might be thinking, *Hey, c'mon, it can't be all that bad. Maybe you just worked with some bad apples.* I have worked with some better apples. Some of my colleagues strive to work with integrity. They are caring, compassionate souls who have a strong work ethic. Unfortunately, I regret to say that some people I have observed in my work have what I would call "god complexes." They feel that their line of work is saving millions of lives, and because of this, they are above reproach. Anyone—not just people in the healthcare industry—can be tempted to idolize him or herself. We often think highly of ourselves and our accomplishments.

To be fair, sometimes pharmaceuticals and other medical treatments do save lives. I am not saying that we should reject every manmade treatment or procedure. My goal is to remind you to put God *first* in everything; before you blindly trust the medical experts, ask God for wisdom and healing.

After asking God for wisdom, you can take a more proactive approach to your health and do your own research. You can go to dailymed.nlm.nih.gov to view drug labels. You can also go to clinicaltrials.gov and find out how different trials are run. Below I'll list some questions worth considering.

HOW TO EVALUATE A CLINICAL TRIAL

- How long has this treatment been studied?

- How many participants were in the study?

- What kind of medical history did the participants have?

- What other drugs were the patients taking while in the study?

- Who was in charge of analyzing the data?

- Who benefits from the results of this study?

- Do I agree with the conclusions that were made from this study?

- Do these studies prove that this treatment is effective?

- Are these studies relevant to me and my specific health needs?

When considering any type of treatment, think of your body as a computer. If you don't take proper care of your computer, it can become overloaded with data and infected by malware. Computers that are overloaded and infected will eventually crash.

In the same way, if we don't take care of ourselves, our bodies will become overloaded with toxins, and we will get sick. If a body is already inundated with excess toxins, one more treatment with harmful ingredients can push that body over the edge. This may happen after one exposure, or maybe it won't happen until the second, third, or five hundredth exposure. You may never even notice any side effects because you and your healthcare provider don't think that a "harmless" treatment could be the main cause of your new ailment.

We should never automatically assume that a manmade treatment is safe for our bodies. Once again, ask the Holy Spirit for wisdom and use that beautiful brain God gave you to do your own research. You may want to consider asking the following questions to help you decide on new medical treatment.

QUESTIONS TO CONSIDER BEFORE UNDERGOING MEDICAL TREATMENT

- How long has this treatment been on the market?

- What are the side effects of this treatment?

- Can my body withstand these side effects?

- Do I see enough evidence that this treatment will be beneficial for my body?

- Do the benefits really outweigh the risks?

You can ask your healthcare provider these questions, but I encourage you to also look for the answers yourself. You can do your own research on pharmaceutical sites, medical device webpages, clinicaltrials.gov, and pubmed.gov. Pubmed.gov contains a plethora of articles from medical journals. It might also be worth your time to connect with in-person or online health support groups to learn about other people's experiences.

There are many respectable healthcare providers; however, they might not have time to take an in-depth approach to your specific case. Some of them are simply following protocols that have been handed to them by healthcare authorities, pharmaceutical companies, and insurance companies. Everybody has unique needs and vulnerabilities. Unfortunately, many medical treatments can cause undue harm to our bodies. But after we have asked God for counsel and have done our due diligence, we will be equipped to make the best decision. It is important to remember that God is all-powerful and that he can also heal us from unwanted side effects. Here's my empowering invitation to you: allow the Holy Spirit to teach you how to be the expert of your own body. The Holy Spirit who lives inside of you will always lead you in the right direction.

If the Drug Stopped the Symptom, My Health Has Improved

"Let no one deceive himself. If anyone among you thinks that he is wise in this age, let him become a fool that he may become wise."

1 CORINTHIANS 3:18

After my sophomore year of college, I transferred to another school that was more appropriate for what I wanted to study. I don't regret that decision, but it was difficult for me to make new friends as a junior at a new school. I was emotionally miserable, grieving over the friends I had left behind, and I was worried about my future.

I'll never forget my last day on campus before graduation. I had probably slept less than four hours the night before, but I woke up feeling elated. *One more final, and then I'm done forever. I can leave this place and go home!* After I took my final, I remember falling over and blacking out for a few seconds as I got out of my car. *Oops, I should've eaten something. Oh well, no time for that. I have to pack up the car so I can get home.*

A few hours later, my small Honda was full of items from my apartment. With very little sleep, food, or water in my system, I started the long drive home. I was so anxious to get home that I didn't even want to stop to go to the bathroom. When I was almost home, I noticed that the low gas indicator on my car was lit up. *I don't want to stop now. I'm almost home!*

Instead of exiting the highway, I pulled over to the side of the road and began to tinker with the gas indicator light (I was probably going bonkers from a lack of food, water, and sleep). *Yes! I was able to turn it off. Off I go.* I didn't get very far. A few miles down the road, my car stopped in the middle of nowhere and it took me hours longer to get home.

Most of this story is true, but the part that involves the gas indicator light is fake. No one would look for a way to turn the gas indicator light off instead of putting gas in the tank. A car is programmed to alert the driver when the car needs gas. In a similar way, God has created gas indicator lights for our bodies. When the body needs extra care, we often experience annoying or distressing symptoms. Unfortunately, instead of giving our bodies what they really need, we often look for a way to turn off the symptom. If the end of this story were actually true and you were a passenger in the car with me, I think that you would surely question my sanity. However, when a person discovers a way to silence their health symptom instead of addressing the actual cause, we normally do not question their logic.

Around 2014, I started developing itchy rashes on my skin. For a while, I used topical steroids to "turn off the symptom." Doctors disagreed on the diagnosis, but a couple of them called it psoriasis.

My symptoms worsened in 2019. What started as dry patches on my fingers eventually progressed to oozing, flaky, painful, itchy rashes that spread to the fronts and backs of my hands. On my worst days, I also had itchy hives on my arms and nasty blotches on my face, neck, underarms, and left foot. When washing dishes, I had to wear cotton gloves under my rubber gloves to avoid additional cuts to my hands. I was afraid to hold my squirmy kids because their clothes irritated my skin whenever they moved around in my arms. At night, I taped a sock to my hand to protect myself from obsessive scratching in my sleep. The worst symptoms lasted from April to December 2019.

About four months after the skin flare started, I discontinued the steroid. I was determined to find out why my skin was so angry. I tweaked my diet several times and visited various alternative health-care practitioners. My skin finally started to clear up after I did a cleanse with essential oils and herbs. My skin was mostly back to normal after I addressed nutritional deficiencies that a functional medicine practitioner found.

Let's play the "What If" game for a second. What if I had only visited a conventional physician and decided to take medications to get rid of the symptoms? In the best-case scenario, my skin would immediately improve with minimal side effects, but my nutrition would continue to decline, leading to additional symptoms and serious disease. In the worst-case scenario, my skin would continue to worsen, and I would need more powerful drugs that cause more serious side effects. My overall health would continue to spiral downward, and I would be left with a pile of medical bills. Turning off the symptom may provide immediate relief, but it is not the wisest plan of action. If you don't give your body what it truly needs, it will eventually stop working.

If I Want to Eliminate My Health Symptoms, I Only Need to Focus on the Physical Needs of My Body

"Heal me, O LORD, and I shall be healed; save me, and I shall be saved, for you are my praise."

JEREMIAH 17:14

Throughout the years, I have learned to recognize the different causes of my abdominal pain. A few months ago, I had to lie down due to abdominal pain and nausea. I knew that the pain was not due to food poisoning, anxiety, or some type of abnormal reaction in my body. I had a feeling that I was being spiritually attacked. I prayed and listened to worship music, and the symptoms were gone in about ten minutes. Doctors are usually not taught to advise their patients to "put on the whole armor of God," but following this advice is crucial for all of us to experience the life that God intended for us. Ephesians 6:10–18 encourages us:

Finally, be strong in the Lord and in the strength of his might. Put on the whole armor of God, that you may be able to stand against the schemes of the devil. For we do not wrestle against flesh and blood, but against the rulers, against the authorities, against the cosmic powers over this present darkness, against the spiritual forces of evil in the heavenly places. Therefore take up the whole armor of God, that you may be able to withstand in the evil day, and having done all, to stand firm. Stand therefore, having fastened on the belt of truth, and having put on the breastplate of righteousness, and, as shoes for your feet, having put on the readiness given by the gospel of peace. In all circumstances take up the shield of faith, with which you can extinguish all the flaming darts of the evil one; and take the helmet of salvation, and the sword of the Spirit, which is the word of God, praying at all times in the Spirit, with all prayer and supplication. To that end, keep alert with all perseverance, making supplication for all the saints.

Our physical bodies are influenced by our souls, other people, the environments around us, the spirit realm, and the Holy Spirit living inside of us. For example, if a person is struggling with depression, there may be numerous factors contributing to her mental and emotional health: she might be experiencing spiritual warfare from demons; she could have unresolved past trauma; she may have abusive relationships; she might have nutritional deficiencies; or she could have toxic mold in her house that is wreaking havoc on all her bodily systems. She could be struggling with depression due to all these above causes. That is why it is necessary to examine the spiritual, mental, social, physical, and environmental aspects of our lives when we are trying to eliminate our symptoms.

It is also beneficial to remember that each part of the physical body is connected to another part; we can't affect one part of the physical body without affecting the whole body. For example, if you experience a sudden, severe injury to the foot, the experience of pain, inflammation, and shock will affect every bodily system—breathing quickens, heart rate goes up, stress hormones are released, muscles become tense, intestinal motility decreases, and anxiety may kick in.

It is also necessary to realize that emotions like fear, grief, resentment, envy, and bitterness can have enormous consequences on our physical health. If we want to experience true, lasting healing, it is crucial to address our spiritual health, negative emotions, and unresolved emotional pain from the past. As Proverbs 14:30 says, "A tranquil heart gives life to the flesh, but envy makes the bones rot."

Many of us know that emotional pain and past trauma can affect our health, but we may not stop to consider that we may be getting sick because of toxins in our environment. This was true of Desiree and Connor. Connor suffered from both indoor and outdoor allergies; his allergies were so severe that he used up a full box of tissues daily. Desiree had grown accustomed to fatigue, digestive issues, and headaches that occurred once or twice per week. The headaches would escalate to migraines and force her to rest in her bed.

Desiree and Connor changed their diets and their health improved. They eventually threw away toxic products (with toxins like phthalates, petrochemicals, carcinogens, and hormone disruptors) in their home and were surprised to see even more positive changes. Desiree shared the following with me:

> My headaches went from one or two times a week to once a month or less. My husband started to breathe better. We both kind of lost that constant "ickiness" in our throats. My husband's allergies massively improved. He stopped going through so many tissues. I think that surprised me because I thought that if I wasn't using something that's chemical and strong enough to kill the bacteria and the germs in my house, I would get sick. That's what they tell us: "If you don't kill the bacteria, you're going to get sick. It's going to get in your body, and you're going to get sick." I was shocked that the opposite happened. My immune system seemed to function better without being exposed to the toxic chemicals that are supposed to be killing things.

Our physical ailments can also be caused by spiritual warfare. As believers in God's word, we know that there is a spiritual realm. However, for whatever reason, sometimes we dismiss the idea that our physical health could be deteriorating due to unseen spiritual attacks. If the "thief comes only to steal and kill and destroy" (John 10:10), it makes sense that the thief would try to destroy our physical bodies.

If you want to improve your health by finding the root cause of your health symptoms, consider acting on the following steps.

FOUR STEPS TO FIND THE ROOT
CAUSE OF YOUR SYMPTOMS

Step 1: Ask God for wisdom and continue asking him for wisdom throughout the process.

Step 2: Ask God to help you evaluate spiritual, mental, social, physical, and environmental impacts on your health. Pick one or more questions from each category below and write some of your uncensored thoughts on a piece of paper. This exercise will help you identify what to focus on.

SPIRITUAL HEALTH

Am I living by the principles in the Bible?
Living according to God's word and his wisdom brings life, peace, and wholeness.

Am I reading and meditating on the Bible?
The Bible can transform our thoughts, actions, and life.

> For the word of God is living and active, sharper than any two-edged sword, piercing to the division of soul and of spirit, of joints and of marrow, and discerning the thoughts and intentions of the heart. (Hebrews 4:12)

Am I spending time with God?
God loves to spend time with us. He wants to be the source of our fulfillment.

> On the last day of the feast, the great day, Jesus stood up and cried out, "If anyone thirsts, let him come to me and drink. Whoever believes in me, as the Scripture has said, 'Out of his heart will flow rivers of living water.'" (John 7:37–38)

Should I consider a fast?

Abstaining from food or another form of comfort (electronics, social media, etc.) can bring us closer to God.

Am I taking time for a Sabbath or a "mini Sabbath"?

God created the Sabbath for our wellness.

> And he said to them, "The Sabbath was made for man, not man for the Sabbath." (Mark 2:27)

Am I trusting in God?

Fear and anxiety are behind many health issues.

Am I rejoicing in God?

Paul found it necessary to tell us to rejoice twice in one sentence.

> Rejoice in the Lord always; again I will say, rejoice. Let your reasonableness be known to everyone. The Lord is at hand. (Philippians 4:4–5)

According to Proverbs, a joyful heart is "good medicine."

> A joyful heart is good medicine, but a crushed spirit dries up the bones. (Proverbs 17:22)

Am I loving God over everything?

Sometimes we don't realize when we prioritize and idolize ourselves, other people, money, fame, power, possessions, dreams, or experiences over God.

> And you shall love the Lord your God with all your heart
> and with all your soul and with all your mind and with
> all your strength. (Mark 12:30)

Have I surrendered all aspects of my life to God?

God knows what is best for us, but we won't receive the best that he has for us unless we give him permission to work in all areas of our lives.

Do I need to "put on the whole armor of God" so that I can "stand against the schemes of the devil"?

> Finally, be strong in the Lord and in the strength of his
> might. Put on the whole armor of God, that you may
> be able to stand against the schemes of the devil. (Ephe-
> sians 6:10–11)

MENTAL HEALTH

Am I focusing on what is true and good?

> Finally, brothers, whatever is true, whatever is honorable,
> whatever is just, whatever is pure, whatever is lovely, what-
> ever is commendable, if there is any excellence, if there
> is anything worthy of praise, think about these things.
> What you have learned and received and heard and seen

in me—practice these things, and the God of peace will
be with you. (Philippians 4:8–9)

Do I need to tweak my schedule so that it reflects the life that God has called me to live?

Our schedules should include time with God, time to take care of our own needs, time for serving others, time for loved ones, time for work, and time for rest.

Am I allowing false beliefs about God, myself, or the world to cloud my thoughts?

Faulty beliefs will result in faulty actions. For example, if you believe that God will shame and condemn you for mistakes that you have made, you might avoid him.

> There is therefore now no condemnation for those who
> are in Christ Jesus. (Romans 8:1)

Am I examining every thought to ensure that it aligns with the Bible?

> We destroy arguments and every lofty opinion raised
> against the knowledge of God, and take every thought
> captive to obey Christ. (2 Corinthians 10:5)

Am I thanking God and telling him my requests?

> Do not be anxious about anything, but in everything
> by prayer and supplication with thanksgiving let your
> requests be made known to God. And the peace of God,

which surpasses all understanding, will guard your hearts and your minds in Christ Jesus. (Philippians 4:6–7)

Do I tend to grumble and argue with others?

Do all things without grumbling or disputing, that you may be blameless and innocent, children of God without blemish in the midst of a crooked and twisted generation, among whom you shine as lights in the world, holding fast to the word of life, so that in the day of Christ I may be proud that I did not run in vain or labor in vain. (Philippians 2:14–16)

Do I need to seek help from God, a mentor, or a professional to heal from trauma?

Some of us don't realize that our lives are deeply affected by abuse, abandonment, or neglect. If we let God heal our wounds, we can walk in freedom from the past.

SOCIAL HEALTH

Do I need to stop isolating myself from other people?

God often uses other people to show us his love.

How has God called me to serve others with my time, money, and gifts?

In all things I have shown you that by working hard in this way we must help the weak and remember the words of the Lord Jesus, how he himself said, "It is more blessed to give than to receive." (Acts 20:35)

Do I spend time with wise people?

There is one whose rash words are like sword thrusts, but the tongue of the wise brings healing. (Proverbs 12:18)

Do not be deceived: "Bad company ruins good morals." (1 Corinthians 15:33)

PHYSICAL HEALTH

Do I need to change my diet?

We might be missing key nutrients in our diets, or we might have to minimize or eliminate certain foods that can cause disease.

Do I move my body on a consistent basis?

Strategic movement will improve circulation in the body, which is beneficial for all parts of the body and mind.

Do I need to change, start, or stop a specific treatment?

The needs of our bodies change over time. It is important to continuously evaluate the benefits and risks of each medication, supplement, or health protocol.

Am I getting enough quality sleep?

Proper rest is imperative for all aspects of health.

Does my body need help with detoxification?

We might experience symptoms when our bodies are overloaded with toxins.

Do I have bowel movements each day or at least every other day?

For optimal health, toxins need to be expelled from the body on a regular basis.

ENVIRONMENTAL HEALTH

Is something in my home causing my health issues or making them worse?

Some examples include excess exposure to electromagnetic frequencies (EMFs), mold, or toxic household and personal care products that interfere with hormones and can cause cancer.

Is something in my neighborhood, school, or workplace making me sick?

A few examples include lack of ventilation, unclean drinking water, and toxic lawn treatment.

Do I need to spend more time in nature?

Science has shown that direct contact with the earth's electrons—a concept called grounding or earthing—can have major health benefits such as improvement in sleep and decreased pain. Sunlight and fresh air are also therapeutic for the body and soul.*

---

* Gaétan Chevalier et al., "Earthing: Health Implications of Reconnecting the Human Body to the Earth's Surface Electrons," *Journal of Environmental and Public Health* (January 12, 2012): https://pubmed.ncbi.nlm.nih.gov/22291721/.

Step 3: Take action.

1. Based on your responses in Step 2, brainstorm and identify one or two simple action steps.

2. Proactively identify any obstacles to success.

3. Create a brief action plan to eliminate possible barriers.

4. Revisit the list of questions in Step 2 every month and ask Holy Spirit to guide you on what to work on next.

Step 4: Look for wise counselors and healthcare professionals (as needed) who can help you find and treat the root cause of your symptoms.

Psychologists, Therapists, Counselors, Coaches, Pastors, or Mentors

Wise mentors who counsel with the wisdom from the Bible and the Holy Spirit can provide invaluable insight and guidance.

Functional Medicine Practitioners

Functional medicine practitioners are medical doctors, registered nurses, nutritionists, and other healthcare professionals who help patients find the root cause of their symptoms. They typically spend several minutes or hours with each patient so that they can create a specific plan for each unique person.

Naturopathic Doctors

A naturopathic doctor works to diagnose, prevent, and treat acute and chronic illness to restore and establish optimal health by supporting the individual's inherent self-healing process. Rather than just suppressing symptoms, naturopathic doctors work to identify underlying causes of illness and develop personalized treatment plans to address them.*

Holistic Health Practitioners and Integrative Health Practitioners

These practitioners evaluate all aspects of health (spiritual, mental, physical, social, and environmental). They treat patients with a combination of conventional and nonconventional forms of therapy.

Chinese Medicine Practitioners

These holistic practitioners use treatments such as acupuncture, herbal remedies, food, movement, and emotional support to promote healing in the body.

Chiropractors

Chiropractors use their hands to manipulate the alignment of the spine and other joints of the body. When the spine is properly aligned, the function of the central nervous system will improve, inflammation will decrease, and the body will be better able to heal itself.

Biological Dentists and Holistic Dentists

Biological dentists provide education for their patients, and they take lifestyle habits, diet, and knowledge of toxicities into consideration. They try to avoid dangerous materials, including amalgam fillings, which contain mercury.

---

* "Home Page," American Association of Naturopathic Physicians, naturopathic.org.

Holistic Optometrists and Ophthalmologists

Holistic optometrists and holistic ophthalmologists evaluate multiple aspects of health (physical, mental, social, and environmental) when caring for their patients' eyes.

Physical Therapists

Physical therapists teach their patients' strategic movements and exercises for pain relief and optimal health. They also provide therapeutic hands-on care.

Massage Therapists

Massage therapists use their hands to manipulate muscles and various parts of the body to provide pain relief, stress relief, and other benefits.

Natural Treatments and Nonconventional Methods Do Not Work

"So Abraham called the name of that place,
'The LORD will provide'; as it is said to this day,
'On the mount of the LORD it shall be provided.'"

GENESIS 22:14

round 2008, a loved one of mine was diagnosed with type 2 diabetes and was told by his endocrinologist that he would have diabetes for the rest of his life—regardless of whether he made lifestyle changes or not. I did not like this response. I am the type of person who doesn't like to be told to just shut up and quit. On a whim, I did an Amazon search for books on treating diabetes naturally. Bingo! Several books popped up. I read the descriptions and the reviews and thought, *Wow. It seems like there are actually people out there who have stopped taking pharmaceuticals and have beaten diabetes with natural methods.* I quickly ordered one of the books. My family member was not interested in changing his health regimen, but reading that book opened my eyes to a growing group of people who were learning how to heal their bodies naturally.

From an early age, I have valued natural solutions over pharmaceuticals. A few years ago, I had an epiphany—I realized why natural solutions work so well. They are effective because God created these methods! For example, he knew that a baby's journey through the birth canal would be beneficial for both the baby's lungs and gut flora. He knew that a formula created by man could never compare to a mom's milk. I find it fascinating that the composition and quantity of breastmilk changes depending on the time of day and the age of the baby. The breastmilk also changes to protect the baby from threats in his specific environment. In the first year of their lives, my three kids were rarely sick, probably because they were receiving "liquid gold" created by God! Breastmilk is not only wonderful for the baby; breastfeeding is greatly beneficial for the mom as well. Some health benefits include mood management, improved sleep, and overall wellness.*

For me, discovering natural remedies is like finding buried treasure. Unfortunately, I've learned that many people do not appreciate them. A few years ago, I was talking to a coworker about natural remedies, and she said something like, "I don't know about natural treatments. The symptoms always come back." I don't remember what I said in response, but when the symptoms on my skin came back, I remembered that conversation. If I were to have the same discussion with her today, I would tell her that sometimes symptoms disappear

---

* Kathleen Kendall-Tackett, Zhen Cong, and Thomas W. Hale, "The Effect of Feeding Method on Sleep Duration, Maternal Well-Being, and Postpartum Depression," *Clinical Lactation* 2, no. 2 (June 2011): https://connect.springerpub.com/content/sgrcl/2/2/22.

forever and sometimes they return, but this happens with both natural and synthetic remedies. I believe that one of the reasons God allows unpleasant symptoms is because they can serve as red flags to show us when something in our life needs to change. For my personal situation, I have noticed that my skin rashes reappear when I am having trouble trusting in God (leading to stress on my mind and body), when I need more time to rest, and when my body is having trouble releasing toxins (this might be due to constipation or another reason).

We experience health symptoms for several reasons, but one of the main causes is that we are not taking proper care of ourselves. In 2010, when my husband and I were trying to buy a house, we visited many houses that were under foreclosure. A few of the houses were dreary, smelly, and dirty. One of them had dead cockroaches under the sink. We also saw a townhouse that looked crooked; it was leaning into the building next to it. As we entered the basement of another house, we were forced to turn around because it was flooded with water!

If we don't want our houses to look like the backdrop of a horror movie, we know that we must maintain them properly. In the same way, if we don't maintain our health, our bodies will start to deteriorate. The upkeep of our homes is rather straightforward, but effective healing of our bodies is not always so. Also, sometimes natural diets and treatments take time to work. We don't always experience instantaneous healing, especially if our bodies have been severely neglected. After years of abuse, the heart, soul, mind, and body might need extra time to heal! It is helpful to remember that if natural treatments do not appear to be effective the first time around, this does not necessarily mean that they do not work for you. Also, remember that every *body* is different. Not every person will benefit from each healthy food, natural remedy, or medication.

Many people claim that there is not enough evidence to confirm that natural remedies are effective. Unfortunately, most clinical trials are performed for synthetic manmade formulations. Money is a huge motivator, and clinical drug research is no exception. Despite a lack of funding on research for natural remedies, pubmed.gov contains countless literature references for natural health treatments. Natural remedies have been used effectively throughout history. Sadly, many people do not believe that they work; therefore, they won't try them, or if they do try them, they will stop using them if they do not notice instant results.

I could write a whole book on natural remedies that work, and there are indeed many books on this topic. I hope that you will be willing to try these amazing tools that God created for our health. And remember, if you decide to try a supplement, herb, essential oil, or any other treatment classified as "natural," seek God's wisdom first, use common sense, and do your own research. Most companies claim that their products are pure, but some of these claims are false.

I have been excited to notice that more people are becoming open to trying natural remedies for health. It is my hope that even more people in our culture would learn about—and embrace—the amazing health benefits of natural foods that are grown and raised the way that God intended. A couple of years ago, I met Eva—a former farmer who told me how God provided healing through natural, grass-fed farming. In her twenties, she was diagnosed with Crohn's disease and was prescribed steroids and sulfa drugs. After several years of symptoms, her health started to spiral downward. In her early forties, she was diagnosed with rheumatoid arthritis. She recounted the following:

> After receiving another prescription of steroids, I sat in my car with my prescription, and I literally cried out to God. I had a big conversation with God, and I said, "I know this is not what you want for me. You do not want me to be dependent on this drug for the rest of my life." Because I knew that I would just get sicker and sicker. I believed in my heart that he had healing in store for me, but I didn't know where to find it. I made a pact with him that I would knock on every door until I found the answer that he had in store for me.

When she went home that day, her husband encouraged her to visit his chiropractor's wife. The chiropractor's wife gave Eva the book *The Body Ecology Diet* by Donna Gates. After three days of following the diet, Eva had no more symptoms of rheumatoid arthritis in her knees. Next, God led Eva to read *The Maker's Diet* by Jordan Rubin. After this, she was introduced to an organic farmer who uses traditional methods to produce unadulterated, nutrient-dense foods.

To be clear, I don't believe our goal should be to avoid synthetic medications at all costs (unless that's what the Holy Spirit is telling you to do). As always, we should ask God for specific instructions on how to take care of our bodies. After we ask God, we may also want to consult with other trusted medical professionals. If you have made God the Lord over your life, I encourage you to make him the Lord over your health as well.

My Body Is Inherently Dysfunctional, and There's Nothing Anyone Can Do About It

"For we are his workmanship, created in Christ Jesus for good works, which God prepared beforehand, that we should walk in them."

EPHESIANS 2:10

remember when I was healthy like you. Then one day I got sick, and it just got worse and worse. Never take your health for granted." My patient was admitted to the hospital with major gastrointestinal issues and pain, had a few tests and intravenous drips, and was sent home. It was the same story every few months—just like other "frequent fliers" on our unit. We saw many patients on a regular basis, but unlike a frequent traveler racking up points, their visits with us were not always useful or rewarding. Some of them did experience brief relief from their symptoms, but the overall status of their health did not seem to improve. The frequent fliers made me wonder, *Do patients ever get better?*

In 2008, that was the question I used to ask myself. I began to believe that just about everyone was predestined to eventually live a life full of physical pain and disease (thankfully, I do not believe this anymore). As time went on, I became very aware of the high number of medical errors that occur in hospitals, and I was afraid of ending up as a frequent flier myself.

Lana shared with me what happened to her mom when she was in the hospital. I could sense that my friend was frustrated. She said, "The doctors want to keep my mom's test result at a certain level, but when they do that, I can tell that it's not good for her. Her memory is becoming very poor, and she is unsteady on her feet. When I told the nurses this, they told me that they agreed with me, but they couldn't change my mom's treatment. If they didn't keep my mom at a certain level, insurance wouldn't cover the treatment."

The medical community has created medical tests, diagnoses, and statistics to attempt to understand and treat disease. A test result or statistic can provide useful information, but we must remember that results and statistics were created by flawed people with biases—all people are flawed and biased—and sometimes conflicts of interest come into play. Patients are diagnosed and misdiagnosed with ailments every day.

When you are given a diagnosis, the healthcare practitioner is merely providing a name for how he or she believes your set of symptoms should be classified. In other words, a diagnosis is simply a word or phrase that reflects your practitioner's understanding of what is going on in your body. Many people plan their medical treatments around the doctor's interpretation. Sometimes people plan their whole lives based upon what the doctor has spoken over them. Placing so much faith in a doctor's judgment can be problematic because these practitioners are far-from-perfect human beings. A test result should not be viewed as a "golden ticket" that provides all the answers that we need. It is also important to note that there is a fair amount of testing that is completely inaccurate. In a perfect world, healthcare decisions would not be determined by unreliable testing and procedures put in place by insurance companies.

There is no shortage of toxins in our world, and our bodies do not function perfectly as God intended them to function. But I believe that God made our bodies much more amazing than we realize. When my children started getting cuts and scrapes, they were so surprised when the skin healed, and the marks disappeared. God designed the body to heal itself! Psalm 139:14 says, "I praise you, for I am fearfully and wonderfully made. Wonderful are your works; my soul knows it very well."

God also created nourishing foods, the earth, soil, sun, plants, and other people for our healing. Genesis 9:3 says, "Every moving thing that lives shall be food for you. And as I gave you the green plants, I give you everything."

It is true that some people are born with certain health challenges that others do not have. The world and the Enemy will try to sell us the "gloom and doom" message that we are powerless over our health. But we are not powerless over our health! We serve the one true God who created the heavens, the earth, and our bodies. Remember that this powerful God who heals the sick, casts out demons, and raises people from the dead—the Holy Spirit—lives inside of you (Romans 8:11)! When Paul was alive, the mere touch of Paul's handkerchief or apron provided healing: "And God was doing extraordinary miracles by the hands of Paul, so that even handkerchiefs or aprons that had touched his skin were carried away to the sick, and their diseases left them and the evil spirits came out of them" (Acts 19:11–12).

I am not saying that this verse automatically means a piece of your clothing will heal a sick person (this could happen, but I am not promising that). I am saying that we are not limited by the laws of this world. God does not want us to be anxious because of our family's genetic history, a test result, or a diagnosis. We serve a supernatural God who has implanted supernatural power inside of us! Nurse Karina experienced God's healing power in her life and she is always excited to share her story with others:

> Whenever we lack wisdom, God invites us to ask him—the One who is omniscient (all-knowing), and true wisdom is given generously. I was healed of 23 years of Chron's disease (a complex, painful autoimmune disease) by nothing but God! When the partial knowledge of humanity—science—told me there was no cure, God said, "I am your healer, follow me." Science and knowledge are gifts from the Almighty One, yet they are not God. Science—when put in its rightful place—helps us, but when we believe the deception that academia, research, and humanity's partial understanding is more powerful than the One who created it all, then it controls us and leaves us susceptible to

more deception. Taste and see that God is good. Do not allow Satan to exploit your pain further. Ask the great I AM to show you his love. He longs to have you close, heal your pain, and give you real power to overcome. Perfect love is victorious.

I want to be clear that it is not my goal to shame or condemn you if you have less-than-ideal health. Regardless of our circumstances, in all aspects of life, God wants us to trust him, expectantly ask him for what we need, and take obedient action. God will take care of the outcome. If you are struggling with physical health symptoms, remember that this all-powerful God who lives inside of you will never leave you or forsake you because you are his child (Hebrews 13:5). Isaiah 41:10 encourages us, "Fear not, for I am with you; be not dismayed, for I am your God; I will strengthen you, I will help you, I will uphold you with my righteous right hand."

I Can Sit Back and Let the Medical System Take Care of Me

"In the thirty-ninth year of his reign Asa was diseased in his feet, and his disease became severe. Yet even in his disease he did not seek the LORD, but sought help from physicians."

2 CHRONICLES 16:12

put a great amount of thought into what I wanted to study in college and what I wanted to do for my career. I knew that I would absolutely hate my job if I didn't feel like I was making a tangible, positive difference in the world. In college, I dabbled in the fields of audiology, law (I wanted to be an attorney to help battered women and children), and social work. I didn't decide on nursing until my aunt set up a meeting with a nurse who worked in a university close to my home. Jackpot! Nursing would provide a flexible, stable career to provide for the kids that I hoped to have someday, and I would be making a real difference in people's lives—I would always be helping people!

Because I had already finished my first bachelor's degree when I decided to become a nurse, I enrolled in a rigorous accelerated nursing program. Nursing school was difficult, but I enjoyed it. When I graduated, I began working on a medical-surgical unit. Some nurses refer to this as the "bedpan unit." We received patients who were sick enough to be hospitalized but not sick enough to be in the intensive care unit. Most days, I felt like all I did was give patients medications and wipe their butts. I wanted to spend more time with the patients and families, but due to the high nurse-patient ratio, that felt impossible. I rushed from one room to another putting out fires, and I was required to spend much of my time "charting"—ensuring that my actions were clearly documented to prove that everything was done right (though I never felt like there was enough time to do anything right!) so that the hospital would not get sued. Follow me as I walk through one of my typical shifts as a bedside nurse.

6:00 p.m.

It's so cold and dark outside. I feel like I haven't seen the sun in a while. I miss the sun. Maybe if I get hit by a car I won't have to go to work. Heh. I'm not going to tell anyone that. If I do, they'll think I'm suicidal. I really need more sleep 'cause three hours is not cutting it. Do they have to schedule a two-hour mandatory training session after the night nurses have already been on their feet for fourteen hours? I don't know how med-surg nurses do this for so many years. I feel like I'm dying.

7:45 p.m.

I just have to get through a couple more of these shifts and then I can sleep. I'll just try to plaster a smile on my face until then. Looks like I have three heavy patients tonight. I have the very loud patient with paranoid schizophrenia in 1218 that threw his bedpan at me yesterday. I also have the 450-pound Mrs. P with a ventilator, urinary catheter, ostomy bag, and stage 3 pressure ulcers. She can't move on her own. I'm going to need help moving her every two hours so that her pressure ulcers don't get worse. The charge nurse gave me the patient in room 1216 with sickle cell disease. He's going to need pain medication every two hours and he will need a new IV line. Is he a hard stick? Last week we had a patient that had to have a line in his foot. I hope Queenie is working tonight to help me.

I also have the man chained to his bed—I wonder what kind of crime he committed. Oh well. Maybe the other three patients will sleep a little bit tonight. I hope that I don't get another admission tonight. The paperwork will take me forever to finish.

11:30 p.m.

Finally done passing out medications. I really need to get some charting done or I will be backed up in the morning. Shoot—1216 wants pain medications and Mrs. P. needs to be changed. Her pressure ulcers can't get worse. I am really not in the mood to be cussed out by her son tonight. It's surprising that 1224 has cancer. She's so young. I wish I had some time to talk to her to see how she is doing.

2:00 a.m. (the next day)

1218 is screaming again. I don't think that his medication is working. If he starts getting violent, security better get here quick.

I can finally get a little bit of charting done. Wait, can't do that yet. Olivia went on break and her patient with Crohn's Disease needs her pain medication. Better give her that medication first and then I have to help Mrs. P before her ostomy bag starts leaking. Gross. I haven't taken a break yet. I really need to pee.

3:30 a.m.

Why is 1216 having trouble breathing? Why am I being paged about 1222? I don't care that he needs a toothbrush right now!

6:00 a.m.

The day shift is going to be here soon. After all the running around that I did tonight, I hope they understand that not everything will be done. I usually stay two hours after my shift to tie up loose ends anyway. I've barely done any charting tonight. That's going to take me a while.

7:00 a.m.

Mrs. P's BP is sky high? Oh, Mrs. P, please don't code on me. Please—hang in there.

1:30 p.m.

Finally in my bed. If someone tries to call me, I will throw my cell phone at the wall.

Unfortunately, healthcare professionals are frequently overworked and over-stressed, and they often don't have enough time to provide the care that each patient needs. Many doctors and healthcare professionals have good intentions; however, as stated before, there are always exceptions. Even doctors with noble intentions can lack wisdom. Wisdom comes from God.

Many people put all their confidence in experts in the healthcare industry. This is not a modern phenomenon. Second Chronicles 16:12 says, "In the thirty-ninth year of his reign Asa was diseased in his feet, and his disease became severe. Yet even in his disease he did not seek the Lord, but sought help from physicians."

Just because many people trust the system, does that make it wise for you to do the same? When facing decisions about your health, I want to encourage you to ask yourself a few important questions: *What is my motivation for agreeing to this treatment or procedure? Am I agreeing to this because the expert told me to do it? Am I agreeing to this because it is a "standard" treatment given to patients when they are diagnosed with this disease? Am I agreeing to it because I have prayed about it, and I feel that the Holy Spirit agrees that this protocol makes the most sense for my particular situation?*

Unfortunately, in our culture of convenience, we tend to outsource our health decisions to the experts with fancy degrees. Have you ever found yourself thinking, *They do the cutting-edge research. They have multiple letters after their names. They went through years and years of schooling that I never went through. They just know better. I am so busy and have so much to do. Why would I waste my time questioning the experts who already have all the answers?* If so, I want to encourage you to pray for wisdom and put that miraculous, intricate brain that God gave you to good use. To put it bluntly—if your brain has been on autopilot because you think that the experts should do your thinking for you, it's time to turn your brain back on!

We are told to follow the doctor's orders. However, if the physician's advice is based solely upon worldly knowledge instead of wisdom from God, should we really expect to see lasting, extravagant results? Jesus came to give us abundant life (John 10:10). He didn't say that we would find abundant life by putting all our hope and trust in doctors.

I am not saying that we should never visit the doctor. In the Bible, Luke was known as a beloved physician (Colossians 4:14). Physicians can provide advice, prescribe treatments, and perform procedures, but it is crucial that we seek God's wisdom *first* in every situation.

For me and my family, we will not say no to every synthetic drug or every manmade procedure, but we are careful about what we say yes to. I went through nursing school, I was a bedside nurse for a short time, and I have worked in the pharmaceutical industry for many years. Unfortunately, my education and experience in the conventional healthcare industry did not teach me how to get healthier—I learned how to thrive outside of that system. You can learn that too—no health degree or science background required. You and God can create a health protocol that works best for *your* body, whether it is inside the healthcare system, outside of it, or a combination of both. *You* are in charge of your health.

Unfortunately, sometimes when we need medical help, we feel too sick to do our own research. When this happens, it is important to have someone who can be an advocate for us. With all three of my pregnancies, I had horrible nausea and vomiting in the first trimester. When I was not working, I spent every free moment in bed because I was overwhelmed with fatigue. I also stayed in the bedroom because the smell of almost any food would push my nausea over the edge. The toilet bowl cleaner smelled like death to me. One evening, after barely tolerating two weeks of nausea and vomiting, I called the on-call doctor. As I expected, he prescribed something for me. I asked him, "Is this safe for the baby?" With noticeable irritation in his voice, he condescendingly answered, "Would I prescribe this to you if the benefits did not outweigh the risks?" If I could have musted up the energy, I would have done my own research, but I felt desperate. I decided to take it. A few days later, I visited my regular doctor, who said, "Do you want to try something else? I would have started you on something gentler. We can try something different."

When I experienced nausea and vomiting with my next pregnancy, I did some research on the treatment that I took with my first baby. At the time of my first pregnancy, the data did not show that there was risk to the child in the womb. At the time of my second pregnancy, animal studies showed a risk to baby animals (meaning the drug was not as safe as previously thought). When I sat down to write this book, I looked for more data. One site says that there is a risk of heart defects, and another site says that the treatment is not recommended for pregnant women living in Australia and the United Kingdom. The manufacturer's label leans toward claiming the drug is "mostly safe for pregnant women," but results are "inconclusive." In the end, I know that God protected us from harm, but this scenario reminds me that I need to be vigilant about what treatments I allow inside my body.

Liliana told me a heartbreaking story of her aunt, who was ninety years old and as "sharp as a tack." Based on her physician's advice, she took a preventive treatment—we will call it "Prophylaxis X"—and after taking it, she did not feel well. She complained of a "fuzzy brain." Later, the physician told her she needed a second round of the treatment. She said that she did not want it, but the doctor told her she had to take it. Right after the treatment, her "mind was gone" and she went blind. She was taken to the hospital for dehydration, and she died soon after. The cause of death written on her death certificate was "Prophylaxis X." This story demonstrates the importance of being an educated advocate for ourselves and our families.

In the gospel of Mark, we read about a woman who had a discharge of blood for twelve years:

> And there was a woman who had had a discharge of blood for twelve years, and who had suffered much under many physicians, and had spent all that she had, and was no better but rather grew worse. She had heard the reports about Jesus and came up behind him in the crowd and touched his garment. For she said, "If I touch even his garments, I will be made well." And immediately the flow of blood dried up, and she felt in her body that she was healed of her disease. And Jesus, perceiving in himself that power had gone out from him, immediately turned about in the crowd and said, "Who touched my garments?" And his disciples said to him, "You see the crowd pressing around you, and yet you say, 'Who touched me?'" And he looked around to see who had done it. But the woman, knowing

what had happened to her, came in fear and trembling and fell down before him and told him the whole truth. And he said to her, "Daughter, your faith has made you well; go in peace, and be healed of your disease." (Mark 5:25–34)

When I first read this story, I was fixated on the discharge of blood and the admirable faith of the woman who touched Jesus' cloak. I read this passage again today with new eyes, and this is what stood out to me: that after seeing many physicians, her health became worse, and she was broke (Mark 5:26).

I have met some notable physicians in my life, and God can use them for good, but we must remember that physicians—even with their degrees and credentials—are not God. They are not the Great Physician. We must not forget the one who created us when it comes to our health. We must always go to God *first* for our health—and for every other aspect of our lives.

As 1 Corinthians 3:18–21 explains, God's wisdom is greater than man's: "Let no one deceive himself. If anyone among you thinks that he is wise in this age, let him become a fool that he may become wise. For the wisdom of this world is folly with God. For it is written, 'He catches the wise in their craftiness,' and again, 'The Lord knows the thoughts of the wise, that they are futile.' So let no one boast in men."

The Bible Has Nothing to Say about My Health

*"All Scripture is breathed out by God and
profitable for teaching, for reproof, for correction,
and for training in righteousness, that the man of God
may be complete, equipped for every good work."*

2 TIMOTHY 3:16-17

Do you ever wish that God provided a mini instruction manual in the Bible for marriage, parenting, or some other area of life? When I searched the Bible for verses related to health, I hoped to find detailed food protocols and other recommendations. I was slightly disappointed that I didn't find much specific information. But as I dug further, I began to realize that a vibrant relationship with Jesus causes a ripple effect in every area of our lives, including our physical health.

Proverbs reveals what can happen when you fear the Lord.

The fear of the LORD is the beginning of wisdom, and the knowledge of the Holy One is insight. For by me your days will be multiplied, and years will be added to your life. (Proverbs 9:10–11)

The fear of the LORD prolongs life, but the years of the wicked will be short. (Proverbs 10:27)

Be not wise in your own eyes; fear the LORD, and turn away from evil. It will be healing to your flesh and refreshment to your bones. (Proverbs 3:7–8)

Is your exhaustion causing health issues? God made the Sabbath to give you rest.

And he said to them, "The Sabbath was made for man, not man for the Sabbath." (Mark 2:27)

Do you have toxic relationships? Ask God to help you find wise friends who will speak life into your soul and body.

Gracious words are like a honeycomb, sweetness to the soul and health to the body. (Proverbs 16:24)

There is one whose rash words are like sword thrusts, but the tongue of the wise brings healing. (Proverbs 12:18)

Peace is life-giving. Envy causes decay.

A tranquil heart gives life to the flesh, but envy makes the bones rot. (Proverbs 14:30)

Rejoicing in the Lord is medicine for your body!

> A joyful heart is good medicine, but a crushed spirit dries
> up the bones. (Proverbs 17:22)

Do not be "dominated by anything."

> "All things are lawful for me," but not all things are help-
> ful. "All things are lawful for me," but I will not be dom-
> inated by anything. (1 Corinthians 6:12)

Your body is for God's glory.

> Or do you not know that your body is a temple of the
> Holy Spirit within you, whom you have from God? You
> are not your own, for you were bought with a price. So
> glorify God in your body. (1 Corinthians 6:19–20)

The word of God provides sustenance and healing.

> But he answered, "It is written, 'Man shall not live by bread
> alone, but by every word that comes from the mouth of
> God.'" (Matthew 4:4)

> My son, be attentive to my words; incline your ear to my
> sayings. Let them not escape from your sight; keep them
> within your heart. For they are life to those who find
> them, and healing to all their flesh. (Proverbs 4:20–22)

In 2019, when I had my worst skin flare accompanied by brain fog,
fatigue, and inflammation, I searched for the "perfect diet" that could

heal my body. I learned that some health experts demonize certain foods while other health gurus confidently label the same a superfood. I was frustrated and confused by what I learned. I eventually avoided so many foods that my weight dropped down to ninety pounds.

I still believe that a healthy diet and a wise health regimen is important for vibrant health. However, I also believe that if a perfect health protocol existed, then God would have written about it in the Bible. The Bible *does* contain content about food, but it does not have an all-extensive list of superfoods and foods to avoid. It does not contain specific information about water intake, carbohydrate counting, or how much exercise someone should aim for in a week.

If we want to consistently measure out our food portions, fill our cabinets with the best health supplements, and engage in daily strenuous exercise, we can certainly do that. Some of our health practices are definitely helpful; however, after all the changes that I have made and after all the research that I have done for my own health, I believe that we will find the most success by walking with God, following simple biblical principles, and listening to the Holy Spirit. I am still mindful about what I put into my body, but I am no longer as legalistic about it as I was before. As I walk on this health journey with God, he continues to show me that true healing—in all aspects—comes from reading his word and from listening to the Holy Spirit. Even though I no longer follow such a stringent diet and health regimen, my overall health (including my physical health) is better than it has ever been.

If you are waiting for healing, remember that God will provide what you need in his perfect timing. He will give you the wisdom that you need, and he will direct your path if you acknowledge him in all your ways:

> And my God will supply every need of yours according to his riches in glory in Christ Jesus. (Philippians 4:19)

> Trust in the Lord with all your heart, and do not lean on your own understanding. In all your ways acknowledge him, and he will make straight your paths. (Proverbs 3:5–6)

PART 2

HOW CAN WE EXPERIENCE TRUE HEALING?

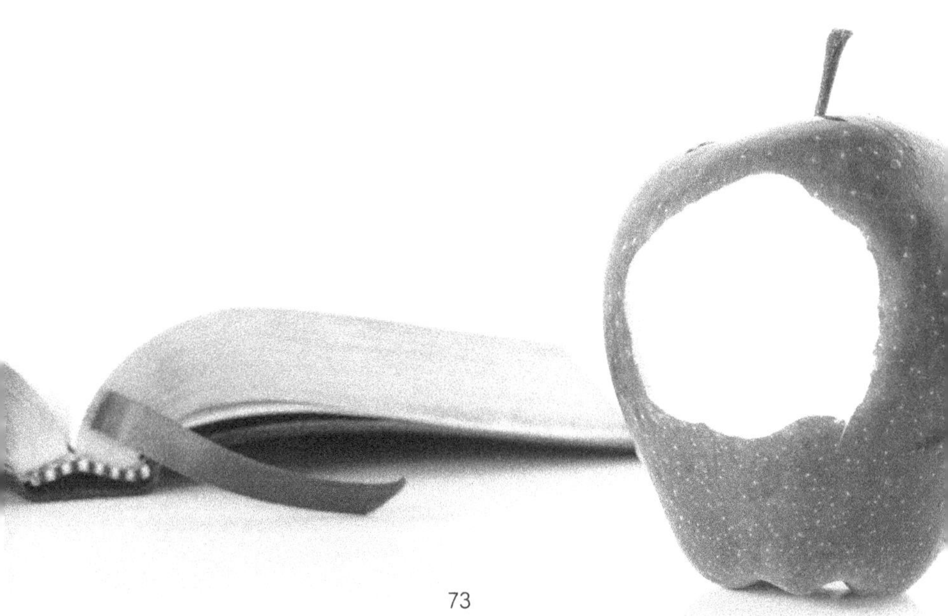

CHAPTER 9

Have Faith and Ask God for Wisdom

"On the way to Jerusalem he was passing along between Samaria and Galilee. And as he entered a village, he was met by ten lepers, who stood at a distance and lifted up their voices, saying, 'Jesus, Master, have mercy on us.' When he saw them he said to them, 'Go and show yourselves to the priests.' And as they went they were cleansed. Then one of them, when he saw that he was healed, turned back, praising God with a loud voice; and he fell on his face at Jesus' feet, giving him thanks. Now he was a Samaritan. Then Jesus answered, 'Were not ten cleansed? Where are the nine? Was no one found to return and give praise to God except this foreigner?' And he said to him, 'Rise and go your way; your faith has made you well.'"

LUKE 17:11-19

n the past, I intentionally followed pastors and teachers from specific Christian denominations. Recently, instead of just believing what others had to say about God, I am exceedingly grateful that God gave me the desire to study the Bible on my own. There are many aspects of God and the Bible that are a mystery to me. I cannot expect to fully understand the maker of heaven and earth. Whether you agree or disagree with what I believe Holy Spirit has revealed to me in his word, my prayer is that you would have an urgent hunger to discover God's incredible truths for yourself.

Evangeline, a friend who experienced pain from fibromyalgia knows what it's like to receive healing from God. She said:

> When I first experienced the fibro pain, I didn't know that it was fibro. Whatever label you want to put on it, it was just constant pain. I was at the point of tears, and I cried out to God, "Please, please, please give me wisdom." The very next day, he showed me that I needed to fast. And I did it. I started eating once a day and the fibro pain was greatly diminished to the point where I felt like I could function again. I share that with you because even if God doesn't heal us instantly like he did when he walked the earth, he can provide wisdom on very simple things that he's provided for us to get better.

I will note that these instructions that Evangeline received are not for everyone who has been diagnosed with fibromyalgia. As previously stated, the Bible says that God will give us wisdom when we ask him for it (James 1:5); therefore, he will give you wisdom for your specific health concern.

The New Testament also contains many stories that display Jesus' power to heal people. We see one example in Matthew 8:5–13:

When he had entered Capernaum, a centurion came forward to him, appealing to him, "Lord, my servant is lying paralyzed at home, suffering terribly." And he said to him, "I will come and heal him." But the centurion replied, "Lord, I am not worthy to have you come under my roof, but only say the word, and my servant will be healed. For I too am a man under authority, with soldiers under me. And I say to one, 'Go,' and he goes, and to another, 'Come,' and he comes, and to my servant, 'Do this,' and he does it." When Jesus heard this, he marveled and said to those who followed him, "Truly, I tell you, with no one in Israel have I found such faith. I tell you, many will come from east and west and recline at table with Abraham, Isaac, and Jacob in the kingdom of heaven, while the sons of the kingdom will be thrown into the outer darkness. In that place there will be weeping and gnashing of teeth." And to the centurion Jesus said, "Go; let it be done for you as you have believed." And the servant was healed at that very moment.

It seems that Jesus was eager to heal the sick people that had faith in him. In contrast, according to Mark 6:5–6, God wanted to do a "mighty work" in his hometown, but he only healed a few people because they did not have faith: "And he could do no mighty work there, except that he laid his hands on a few sick people and healed them. And he marveled because of their unbelief."

When my daughter had ongoing health issues, I persistently searched for answers. I remembered a book that a friend recommended to me entitled *God's Medicine Bottle* by Derek Prince. After I read it the second time, one Bible passage came alive to me: "My son, be attentive to my words; incline your ear to my sayings. Let them not escape from your sight; keep them within your heart. For they are life to those who find them, and healing to all their flesh" (Proverbs 4:20–22).

God's words are healing to the flesh! Using Psalm 91, *Prayers & Proclamations* by Derek Prince (prayers and proclamations from the Bible), and other Bible resources, I boldly and expectantly began praying Scripture over my daughter three times per day, just like medicine. On one day, after starting this practice, she had a fever and became increasingly fatigued. As she was drifting off to sleep, I prayed Scripture over her again. I had not given her any fever reducers, essential oils, or supplements, but her fever was gone after I prayed. The next day, when her fever came back, I prayed Scripture over her again. Immediately after I prayed, the fever was gone. God has also instantaneously healed coughs and tummy aches that my children have had.

I do not have all the answers when it comes to faith and healing. Jesus healed many people in the New Testament. However, we also see that God did not take Paul's "thorn in the flesh" away (2 Corinthians 12). Some theologians believe that Paul's thorn was a physical ailment, while others believe that it was persecution from others or something else. We may never know why some people are healed and some are not healed, but if we read the Bible, we can't deny that God moves mightily when his people have tremendous faith. This begs the question: How can we increase our faith?

Read the Bible.

> So faith comes from hearing, and hearing through the word of Christ. (Romans 10:17)

Don't follow the world. "Be transformed by the renewal of your mind."

> Do not be conformed to this world, but be transformed by the renewal of your mind, that by testing you may discern what is the will of God, what is good and acceptable and perfect. (Romans 12:2)

"Be doers of the word."

> But be doers of the word, and not hearers only, deceiving yourselves. (James 1:22)

Remember what God has already done.

> I will remember the deeds of the Lord; yes, I will remember your wonders of old. I will ponder all your work, and meditate on your mighty deeds. (Psalm 77:11–12)

Ask God for more faith.

> The apostles said to the Lord, "Increase our faith!" And the Lord said, "If you had faith like a grain of mustard seed, you could say to this mulberry tree, 'Be uprooted and planted in the sea,' and it would obey you." (Luke 17:5–6)

And Jesus said to him, "'If you can'! All things are possible for one who believes." Immediately the father of the child cried out and said, "I believe; help my unbelief!" And when Jesus saw that a crowd came running together, he rebuked the unclean spirit, saying to it, "You mute and deaf spirit, I command you, come out of him and never enter him again." And after crying out and convulsing him terribly, it came out, and the boy was like a corpse, so that most of them said, "He is dead." But Jesus took him by the hand and lifted him up, and he arose. (Mark 9:23-27)

Sometimes God allows trials so that we will become mature and complete, lacking in nothing (James 1:2–4). Sometimes God allows hardship to keep us humble; he wants to teach us that his grace is sufficient for us (2 Corinthians 12:7–10). As previously stated, in 2 Corinthians 12, Paul pleaded with God about a thorn in his flesh, but God did not remove the thorn. Therefore, if God does not take away our "thorns"—whatever those are for us—we can remember that God has a purpose for the suffering, and we can ask him to help us trust him with that purpose. We can trust in the one who has already proven that he loves us with a steadfast love.

I have been blessed to know Luisa, a Christian life coach who allowed God to turn her suffering into a thriving ministry. In her words, she was a normal, boring stay-at-home mom who sent her kids to private Christian school. Her husband often traveled for work.

One night, while her husband was away, there was a knock on the door. She opened the door to a man standing on her doorstep. There was also a woman in the driveway. The man proceeded to tell her that her husband owed him money. In a few seconds, she came to realize that the man standing at her door was a pimp and the woman in the driveway was a prostitute her husband had been with. This "normal" stay-at-home mom had no idea that her husband was leading a double life.

As she reluctantly trudged through counseling, she was angry at God. She didn't understand why God had never given her a hint about her husband's infidelity and deception. She told me, "I made God a promise that if he ever got me out of the living hell that I was in, then I would spend the rest of my life teaching others how to get out." God blessed her with another woman who walked with her as she healed from the trauma of what happened in her marriage. God ultimately provided healing and restoration for her marriage as well.

Luisa has spent the last twelve years helping men and women heal from trauma and emotional pain. Her story will always be a reminder to me of how God can transform our stories of profound pain into stunning demonstrations of beauty, restoration, and hope that will affect future generations for eternity.

In addition to having faith, we need to have humility and ask God for his advice. An account from the book of Joshua contains a significant lesson for us. If you do an internet search for information on Joshua in the Bible, you'll find descriptions such as "divine warrior," "the greatest military leader of all time," and "man of faith." Joshua was known as an exceptional leader. However, after reading all these honorable nicknames for Joshua, you may be surprised to find that he was deceived by the Gibeonites because he "did not ask counsel from the LORD" (Joshua 9:14).

Some of us believe that God will automatically stop us from making a mistake. The Bible has examples of what God will do to capture a person's attention. He opens the mouths of donkeys (Numbers 22), instructs big fish to capture runaways (Jonah 1), and provides specific commands in dreams (Matthew 1). However, as we can see in Joshua 9, God does not always intervene. Unfortunately, the truth is that we can be deceived about issues regarding our health, money, vocation, relationships, and any other aspect of our lives. We may spend our whole lives being deceived about certain issues if we don't ask God for his counsel.

I am not sure why Joshua did not ask God for advice, but I can think of reasons why we might avoid seeking counsel from him. Perhaps we don't really believe that God cares about us or the details of our lives. If we study the microscopic parts of a plant, animal, or human, we will quickly realize how creative and detail-oriented God is. The Bible says that the hairs of our head are all numbered (Luke 12:7)! I believe that this meticulous God cares deeply about the details of our lives.

We may want to surrender every part of our lives to God, but some of us are too distracted to realize that we are placing other priorities before him. We are unaware of the ways we are not allowing him to work in our lives. And because we are so distracted, we don't notice God's warnings, instructions, or blessings.

Maybe we don't ask God for his counsel because we don't think we will get a clear answer from him. God does not usually speak audibly to us, but the Bible says that God rewards those who seek him. He will provide us with wisdom in his own way and in his own timing. Hebrews 11:6 says, "And without faith it is impossible to please him, for whoever would draw near to God must believe that he exists and that he rewards those who seek him."

A friend of mine reminded me of James 5 when I was struggling with my health. I am grateful to the pastor of my church who prayed over me and anointed my head with oil. Also, confessing my sins to other sisters in Christ has provided healing in many areas of my life. James 5 says:

> Is anyone among you suffering? Let him pray. Is anyone cheerful? Let him sing praise. Is anyone among you sick? Let him call for the elders of the church, and let them pray over him, anointing him with oil in the name of the Lord. And the prayer of faith will save the one who is sick, and the Lord will raise him up. And if he has committed sins, he will be forgiven. Therefore, confess your sins to one another and pray for one another, that you may be healed. The prayer of a righteous person has great power as it is working. (James 5:13–16)

Jesus said that we would have tribulation in this life (John 16:33). He also said, "If anyone would come after me, let him deny himself and take up his cross and follow me" (Matthew 16:24). I used to believe that these two passages meant that following God leads to a life of misery. I no longer believe this to be true. You have probably heard this phrase about God over and over again: "He's a good Father." But do you truly believe it?

I believe that God wants us to ask him for good gifts, and he wants to give us good gifts.

> If you then, who are evil, know how to give good gifts to your children, how much more will your Father who is in heaven give good things to those who ask him! (Matthew 7:11)

I believe that if we delight in his righteousness, God delights in our welfare. The dictionary defines *welfare* as well-being, happiness, or prosperity.

> Let those who delight in my righteousness shout for joy and be glad and say evermore, "Great is the LORD, who delights in the welfare of his servant!" (Psalm 35:27)

I believe that God wants us to experience his goodness while we are on this earth.

> I believe that I shall look upon the goodness of the LORD in the land of the living! Wait for the LORD; be strong, and let your heart take courage; wait for the LORD! (Psalm 27:13–14)

I believe that God wants us to experience some of heaven on earth. Why else would Jesus tell us to pray that his will be done on earth as it is in heaven?

> Pray then like this: "Our Father in heaven, hallowed be your name. Your kingdom come, your will be done, on earth as it is in heaven." (Matthew 6:9–10)

I believe that the lies and twisted passions of the world will enslave us. God wants to give us rest, and the burden that God calls us to carry is light.

> Come to me, all who labor and are heavy laden, and I will give you rest. Take my yoke upon you, and learn from me, for I am gentle and lowly in heart, and you will find rest for your souls. For my yoke is easy, and my burden is light. (Matthew 11:28–30)

I pray that these truths would penetrate our hearts. If we don't believe that God is a good Father who wants to give us good gifts, then we probably won't ask him for what we want or need. Jesus' sacrifice allowed us to approach God with boldness (Hebrews 10:19)! I pray that we would fully understand how extravagantly blessed we are.

CHAPTER 10

Know the Truth and Meditate on the Truth

*"If you abide in my word, you are truly my disciples, and
you will know the truth, and the truth will set you free."*

JOHN 8:31-32

Because I grew up in the church, I thought I knew all there was
to know about God. And yet, at the same time, the Bible was
often confusing or boring to me. In 2016, God placed inspiring people in my life who woke me up to what I was missing. After
joining a women's group in my church, I saw the gradual transformation of many of the ladies around me. One of them mentioned
that she couldn't get enough of the Bible. She read it all the time.
Another friend carried her Bible around everywhere she went. She
would say, "You never know when you're going to need it." I was so
intrigued by their love for God's word. I wondered, *Why don't I feel
that way about the Bible?*

Around the same time, a friend of mine posted a suggestion on Facebook that caught my attention: "If you don't love the Bible, just pray and ask God to help you love it." I started asking God this simple request. About a year later, I realized that God was answering that prayer—I started to understand the Bible more and I began to love the transformational truths that I was learning. If you want to love the Bible and love God more each day, tell your heavenly Father about this desire. He will answer this prayer! James 4:8 says, "Draw near to God, and he will draw near to you." And John 14:13–14 says, "Whatever you ask in my name, this I will do, that the Father may be glorified in the Son. If you ask me anything in my name, I will do it."

The Bible began to set me free from the lies that I had believed about God, the world, and myself. We are constantly bombarded by subtle variations of the truth. It is vital that we continually immerse ourselves in God's word—the truth that sets us free—so that we do not become "slaves" to these subtle lies in our culture (Galatians 5:1).

Some of us might not seek God's wisdom in the Bible because we are afraid of what we will learn. Maybe we do not fully surrender every part of our lives to God because his way seems strange, unpopular, or difficult. When we feel insecure, we need to remember who we serve:

The Living God (Joshua 3:10)

Our Refuge (Psalm 62:8)

My Helper (Psalm 54:4)

The Most High God (Daniel 3:26)

The Faithful God (Deuteronomy 7:9)

God at Hand (Jeremiah 23:23)

My Salvation (Psalm 51:14)

God of Seeing (Genesis 16:13)

My Exceeding Joy (Psalm 43:4)

A Consuming Fire (Deuteronomy 4:24)

The Lord, Mighty in Battle (Psalm 24:8)

Provider (Genesis 22:14)

My Rock, My Fortress, My Deliverer, My Stronghold (Psalm 18:2)

My Shepherd (Psalm 23:1)

Your Healer (Exodus 15:26)

Wonderful Counselor, Mighty God, Everlasting Father, Prince of Peace (Isaiah 9:6)

Light for the Nations (Isaiah 42:6)

I AM (Exodus 3:14)

If we are feeling insecure, it is also empowering to remember who we are because of Christ:

Blessed with every spiritual blessing in the heavenly places (Ephesians 1:3)

Chosen (Ephesians 1:4)

Adopted by God (Ephesians 1:5)

Redeemed and forgiven (Ephesians 1:7)

Sealed with the promised Holy Spirit, who is the guarantee of our inheritance (Ephesians 1:13–14)

Precious (1 Peter 2:4)

Chosen race, royal priesthood, holy nation, people for his own possession (1 Peter 2:9)

One of God's people that has received mercy (1 Peter 2:10)

Sojourner (1 Peter 2:11)

Salt of the earth (Matthew 5:13)

Light of the world (Matthew 5:14)

Fearfully and wonderfully made (Psalm 139:14)

In John 14:12, Jesus himself also said, "Truly, truly, I say to you, whoever believes in me will also do the works that I do; and greater works than these will he do, because I am going to the Father." Notice that Jesus said *truly* twice, and notice that he used the word *whoever.* Jesus wants you to *truly* know that you have the authority to do the *powerful* works that he did. The "Spirit of him who raised Jesus from the dead dwells in you" (Romans 8:11)!

I want to encourage you to keep these truths and other biblical truths in a note on your phone, in your journal, and on your refrigerator. Post the truth everywhere! After Luisa found out about her husband's involvement with prostitutes, she clung to the word of God as her lifeline. She placed countless Post-it notes all over her walls. Her young kids noticed how the small yellow scraps of paper were helping their mom, so when they saw the Post-it notes fall to the floor, they scrambled to tape them back on the wall so that their mom could feel okay again.

When I was younger, it would only take one negative comment from someone, one small setback in my day, one unwelcome thought, or one piece of bad news to send my mind spiraling into confusion, anxiety, or depression. I was taught to meditate on God's word at all times, but I did not understand—or believe—the impact that it could have on my life. The Bible is the sword of the Spirit (Ephesians 6:17), a weapon that we must use against lies and the darkness. The devil tried to tempt Jesus when he was vulnerable, but he gave up after Jesus fought back with powerful truth from the word of God:

> Then Jesus was led up by the Spirit into the wilderness to be tempted by the devil. And after fasting forty days and forty nights, he was hungry. And the tempter came and said to him, "If you are the Son of God, command these stones to become loaves of bread." But he answered, "It is written,
>
> "'Man shall not live by bread alone,
>> but by every word that comes from the
>> mouth of God.'"
>
> Then the devil took him to the holy city and set him on the pinnacle of the temple and said to him, "If you are the Son of God, throw yourself down, for it is written,

"'He will command his angels concerning you,'

and

"'On their hands they will bear you up,
    lest you strike your foot against a stone.'"

Jesus said to him, "Again it is written, 'You shall not put the Lord your God to the test.'" Again, the devil took him to a very high mountain and showed him all the kingdoms of the world and their glory. And he said to him, "All these I will give you, if you will fall down and worship me." Then Jesus said to him, "Be gone, Satan! For it is written,

"'You shall worship the Lord your God
    and him only shall you serve.'"

Then the devil left him, and behold, angels came and were ministering to him. (Matthew 4:1–11)

If we want healthy souls that can lead to healthy bodies, success, joy, and peace, it is crucial to keep our minds on God's truth throughout the *entire* day.

Only be strong and very courageous, being careful to do according to all the law that Moses my servant commanded you. Do not turn from it to the right hand or to the left, that you may have good success wherever you go. This Book of the Law shall not depart from your mouth, but you shall meditate on it day and night, so that you may be careful to do according to all that is written in it. For then you will make your way prosperous, and then you will have good success. (Joshua 1:7–8)

You keep him in perfect peace whose mind is stayed on you, because he trusts in you. (Isaiah 26:3)

Set your minds on things that are above, not on things that are on earth. (Colossians 3:2)

For though we walk in the flesh, we are not waging war according to the flesh. For the weapons of our warfare are not of the flesh but have divine power to destroy strongholds. We destroy arguments and every lofty opinion raised against the knowledge of God, and take every thought captive to obey Christ. (2 Corinthians 10:3-5)

CHAPTER 11

Pray for a Change of Heart, Ears to Hear, and Eyes to See

"For this people's heart has grown dull, and with their ears they can barely hear, and their eyes they have closed, lest they should see with their eyes and hear with their ears and understand with their heart and turn, and I would heal them." But blessed are your eyes, for they see, and your ears, for they hear. For truly, I say to you, many prophets and righteous people longed to see what you see, and did not see it, and to hear what you hear, and did not hear it."

MATTHEW 13:15-17

When I was struggling with resentment and unforgiveness, a friend of mine encouraged me to ask God to change my heart. David expresses this desire in Psalm 139:23–24, which says, "Search me, O God, and know my heart! Try me and know my thoughts! And see if there be any grievous way in me, and lead me in the way everlasting!" Ever since I started asking God to change my heart, I feel as if my capacity to sense God's love and healing power has increased.

God wants to provide us with wisdom for every aspect of our lives, but sometimes we cannot hear what God is saying to us because our hearts have "grown dull" (Matthew 13:15). As stated before, the state of our physical health is dependent upon various factors. Our physical bodies are affected by our physical health practices (food choices, medications, exercise, etc.), spiritual health, mental health, relationships, and environment. Therefore, if we desire God's wisdom for all these areas of our lives, our hearts need transformation so that we can see what God wants us to see and hear what God wants us to hear.

I can think of four specific times when I was certain that I heard the voice of God. His voice was unmistakable and wonderfully overwhelming. I didn't hear an audible voice, but I knew that God was speaking to me.

My previous church had a time of prayer and fasting at the beginning of each year. Around 2016, instead of fasting from food, I decided to fast from TV. Back then, I was accustomed to watching hours of TV whenever I had free time. On a dreary Sunday afternoon when I was fasting, I felt depressed, and I decided to lie down on the bed. After about fifteen minutes, a thought popped into my head from out of nowhere: *You think that I love other people more than I love you because you think that their lives are easier than yours.* My eyes popped open. I was dazed and bewildered. I thought, *God? Why did you say that?*

After a few days of reflection, I knew why he said it to me. I felt entitled to my definition of an ideal life. When I couldn't instantaneously attain "the next best thing," I decided to believe the lie that God is unfair, and I chose to believe that God loved other people more than he loved me. The truth is, because of Jesus' sacrifice for me, I have everything that I need. I also have an inheritance—an eternity of unimaginable pleasures and joy with God. David declares in Psalm 16:11, "You make known to me the path of life; in your presence there is fullness of joy; at your right hand are pleasures forevermore."

James 1:2–4 teaches us the truth that God allows temporary trials in our lives so that we can grow: "Count it all joy, my brothers, when you meet trials of various kinds, for you know that the testing of your faith produces steadfastness. And let steadfastness have its full effect, that you may be perfect and complete, lacking in nothing."

If I had not decided to take a break from TV, I probably would have missed what God wanted to tell me. It is also worth noting that God is a jealous god; he didn't welcome the fact that I was constantly placing TV, other people, and other priorities before him. Exodus 34:14 instructs us, "For you shall worship no other god, for the LORD, whose name is Jealous, is a jealous God."

I distinctly remember another time God's gentle voice interrupted my destructive thoughts and worries. I had been dreading a particular event for a couple of months and felt as if I had an unrelenting raincloud over my head. It was a cold and dreary day in Chicago. I dragged my feet down into my basement and picked up a basket of laundry. An unexpected thought tenderly pierced through my melancholic numbness: *You know that I will be with you, right?*

And I will never forget the encounter I had with God after I asked him for advice on whether I should move to a different state. In the middle of another bitter winter in Chicago, in 2020, I jokingly said to my husband, "Hey, maybe we should move to Florida." For whatever reason, I thought he disliked Florida and would never consider moving there. We had also previously decided that it would be foolish for us to move away from all the friends and family who surrounded us in Chicago. Despite our previous decision, to my surprise, my husband did not seem to hate the idea of moving to Florida.

Early in 2021, after our landlord kicked us out of her house, we were forced to make a quick decision on where to move next. After hours of research and prayer, my husband and I decided to make a quick two-night trip to Florida to scope out the area. Before I left, I asked people to pray for us. Despite all the research and discussions with my husband, I was almost 100 percent sure that we would not move. In my mind, we were making a fun, quick exploratory trip, and then we would return to our regular routine. Ever since I was a kid, I've detested the cold and longed for something different, but the thought of leaving practically every single loved one behind felt scary and foreign.

On the second and last day we were there, I decided to rest on a hammock before the sun went down. The warm air felt glorious— a brief, welcome escape from the harsh winter temperatures that I had unenthusiastically grown accustomed to over the years. Before I explain what happened, I want to assure you that I was fully sober; not a drop of alcohol or any other mind-altering substance had entered my body. I was reading a prayer book that had verses written in each chapter, and I came across a verse that I had read a couple times in the past.

As I read the verse, I felt the atmosphere around me start to spin. I quickly sat up. I looked at the houses across the street, the trees, the grass, the hammock, and my hands—everything was blurry. I gazed down at the page in front of me and realized that the only thing I could see clearly was the verse written there. I read the verse two more times. After about fifteen seconds, the spinning stopped, and my vision returned to normal.

After living in Florida for almost two years now, I look back on that experience and know that God spoke to me through that one Bible verse; he used that verse to tell me that he wanted us to move away from Chicago.

I will never forget how God spoke to me and my children in 2022 when Hurricane Ian hit Florida. When it was clear that the hurricane was going to hit our area, I was not anxious until I realized how massive the storm was. On the day of the hurricane, I was listening to a podcaster talk about how she taught her kids to hear God's voice. I was trying to pay some bills, but I felt my anxiety start to rise. I couldn't focus. I went downstairs and asked the kids to sit around the table.

I prayed, "Hi, God. We just want to hear from you. Do you have something to tell us? Will you speak to us?"

After a few minutes, I asked the kids, "Did you hear anything from God?"

My four-year-old son quietly replied, "Yes, I did."

I asked, "What did you hear?"

My four-year-old answered, "I will protect you."

I told the kids, "I heard something too. I heard, 'Don't be scared' and 'I'm happy to talk with you.'"

I wish that God always spoke to me that clearly, and there are times when I am frustrated by the fact that it can be difficult to know when God is trying to tell me something. I think that I would gladly welcome conversations with God via burning bushes (Exodus 3) or angels (Luke 1). Though I will never fully understand God, I know that the Bible describes him as my Father, husband, and friend:

> If you then, who are evil, know how to give good gifts to your children, how much more will your Father who is in heaven give good things to those who ask him! (Matthew 7:11)

> For your Maker is your husband, the LORD of hosts is his name; and the Holy One of Israel is your Redeemer, the God of the whole earth he is called. (Isaiah 54:5)

> No longer do I call you servants, for the servant does not know what his master is doing; but I have called you friends, for all that I have heard from my Father I have made known to you. (John 15:15)

I will not know my earthly father, earthly husband, or earthly friends intimately unless I make a continuous, intentional effort to do so. Intimacy, depth, and understanding in a relationship is not easily obtained. It's the same with God. I will not be able to understand God on a deeper level unless I read the Bible and communicate with him. On some days, I get frustrated because I feel like I don't understand God—especially when it seems like I can't hear him clearly. On other days, I am humbly overwhelmed and grateful by the fact that the kind, mysterious maker of heaven and earth would speak to me at all!

God speaks to his people in various ways. He speaks to us through the Bible, thoughts in our head, music, circumstances, visions, dreams, people, and other mysterious ways. He will never give us guidance that conflicts with the Bible. We tend to forget that God's written word is one of the primary ways that we can hear directly from him. When we are reading this beautiful ancient text, we are reading God's very words spoken to us. As John 1:1 says, "In the beginning was the Word, and the Word was with God, and the Word was God."

God often speaks directly into my specific situation through his word, and his word helps me see the world through an accurate lens. More importantly, reading the Bible helps me know God more intimately. The more we read the Bible, the more we will know God's voice. The more we know his voice, the less likely we are to be deceived by all the other voices that want to distract or harm us. Jesus tells us in John 10:27–28, "My sheep hear my voice, and I know them, and they follow me. I give them eternal life, and they will never perish, and no one will snatch them out of my hand."

My children went through a period of time when they had detailed, disturbing nightmares. I started teaching them how to call to Jesus for help when they needed him. My seven-year-old daughter came to me the other day and told me that she had a nightmare. In her dream, she was being pursued by an attacker. She ran into her brother's room and cowered in the corner. She yelled out, "Help me, Jesus! Help me, Jesus!" She saw light and there was wind. A spark appeared in her hand that turned into a pear.

My eyes began to widen as she spoke. I became increasingly excited as I realized what her dream meant. Jesus is the light of the world (John 8:12) and the Holy Spirit ascended from heaven with a "sound like a mighty rushing wind" in Acts 2:2. Jesus and Holy Spirit appeared to my daughter in her dream! I told her, "Let's ask God why he gave you a pear." She replied, "He gave me a pear to show me that he's here for me and to show me that he loves me. He knows I love pears. There was a heart on the pear."

A few months ago, my daughter saw an angel in the backyard. She told me, "The angel was there because I was scared. He stayed there until I fell asleep." When I told my friend this story, she reminded me of Psalm 91:11, which says, "For he will command his angels concerning you to guard you in all your ways." I praise God for protecting my family!

I can also see how God is training my eleven-year-old daughter to trust in his word. She asks me thought-provoking questions that help grow my own faith, and she reads the Bible daily. God's word is constantly being fulfilled in our lives. I pray that we would have hearts of flesh, ears to hear, and eyes to see God's healing work all around us. May we have the hearts that God promised to give his people in Ezekiel 36:26, "And I will give you a new heart, and a new spirit I will put within you. And I will remove the heart of stone from your flesh and give you a heart of flesh."

CHAPTER 12

Be Obedient and Trust God with the Outcome

*"And he cried to the LORD, and the LORD showed him a
log, and he threw it into the water, and the water became
sweet. There the LORD made for them a statute and a rule, and
there he tested them, saying, 'If you will diligently listen to
the voice of the LORD your God, and do that which is right
in his eyes, and give ear to his commandments and keep
all his statutes, I will put none of the diseases on you that I
put on the Egyptians, for I am the LORD, your healer.'"*

EXODUS 15:25-26

Sometimes we know how to improve our health, or God has already told us what to do, but we don't want to obey his instruction. In 2 Kings 5, before Naaman was healed, he "went away in a rage":

And Elisha sent a messenger to him, saying, "Go and wash in the Jordan seven times, and your flesh shall be restored, and you shall be clean." But Naaman was angry and went away, saying, "Behold, I thought that he would surely come out to me and stand and call upon the name of the LORD his God, and wave his hand over the place and cure the leper. Are not Abana and Pharpar, the rivers of Damascus, better than all the waters of Israel? Could I not wash in them and be clean?" So he turned and went away in a rage. But his servants came near and said to him, "My father, it is a great word the prophet has spoken to you; will you not do it? Has he actually said to you, 'Wash, and be clean'?" So he went down and dipped himself seven times in the Jordan, according to the word of the man of God, and his flesh was restored like the flesh of a little child, and he was clean. (2 Kings 5:10–14)

If we engage in unhealthy habits, we may already know that our excess junk food, stressful schedules, or lifestyle choices are causing our health to fail. We may know that this is true for us, but some of us do not take the necessary steps for change. Our bodies are temples of the Holy Spirit (1 Corinthians 6:19), and I believe that God wants us to take proper care of these temples. God will show us what we need to know—all we need to do is ask for his help. God might also provide coaches, mentors, and friends to train us and keep us accountable. God calls us to obedience. He also asks us to trust him with the outcome of our obedient actions: "Blessed is the man who trusts in the LORD, whose trust is the LORD. He is like a tree planted by water, that sends out its roots by the stream, and does not fear when heat comes, for its leaves remain green, and is not anxious in the year of drought, for it does not cease to bear fruit" (Jeremiah 17:7–8).

The above passage in Jeremiah paints such a beautiful word picture of spiritual health. Earlier this year, when I had painful rashes on my skin, I followed my regular health protocols that worked in the past. I consumed healing foods and remedies and visited a naturopathic doctor. My skin improved a bit, but only for a short period of time. I asked God what to do next. When I saw this Bible passage in a few different places, I sensed God was showing me that my lack of trust in him was contributing to my symptoms. Sometimes my skin mirrors what is going on inside my mind. When I lack trust in God, I become anxious. This anxiety triggers inflammation in my body, and the inflammation leads to "angry" skin.

Sometimes I can see my health symptoms as a blessing. Instead of letting my mind and body spiral further down the path of anxiety and inflammation, God allows these symptoms so that I know when I need to focus on my physical health and when I need to rely more on him. A lack of trust in God may not be the reason for your health symptoms, but I believe that this is true in my situation.

When I am having a difficult time trusting in God, it helps to remember the life that Jesus lived and the sacrifice that he made. This all-powerful God was placed in a manger (a feeding trough!). This King of kings allowed deceived, self-obsessed humans to spit on him, ridicule him, torture him, and nail him to a cross. This Most High God—the creator of heaven and earth—created trees and allowed thorns on vines. Before humans even existed, God knew that he would one day be falsely accused, brutally abused, and nailed to one of the trees that he created. He also knew that the thorns on the vines that he created would one day be used as a disgraceful tool of mockery and pain on his very own head. He knew that we would constantly place other "gods" before him, but he still chose humility, mockery, and torture for himself—so that we could have freedom and everlasting life with him. Let us realize and never forget that Jesus did not have to say yes to any of this. He could have simply destroyed us. Jesus' sacrifice provides the true definition of love for us: "Greater love has no one than this, that someone lay down his life for his friends" (John 15:13).

When we have trouble trusting in God, we can meditate on the truth that God loves us with a love that is completely pure, faithful, never-ending, and trustworthy. This all-powerful, supernatural, loving God asks us to trust him, regardless of the outcome.

God never promised us an easy life (John 16:33), and as far as our health is concerned, we may struggle with pain and other symptoms. But God will never leave us or forsake us (Hebrews 13:5). And he does promise to use all the difficulty in our lives for good: "And we know that for those who love God all things work together for good, for those who are called according to his purpose" (Romans 8:28). God desires to be everything to us, not only because he loves us with a fierce, perfect, unexplainable love, but because he knows that an intimate connection with him is what will give us the abundant life we were made for.

If Jesus is the Lord of our lives, then he is the Lord of our bodies and health. If we continue to seek God and ask the Holy Spirit for wisdom, we can trust that he will give us the wisdom to take care of the bodies he created. God's grace is sufficient for us (2 Corinthians 12:9). If a cloud of depression causes a seemingly never-ending spiral of irritation, numbness, and brain fog; if your rambunctious two-year-old is suddenly diagnosed with a debilitating illness; if your best friend receives a disturbing report from the doctor, are you willing to turn to God *first* for comfort, counsel, and healing? Jesus calls to us, "Come to me, all who labor and are heavy laden, and I will give you rest. Take my yoke upon you, and learn from me, for I am gentle and lowly in heart, and you will find rest for your souls. For my yoke is easy, and my burden is light" (Matthew 11:28–30).

ABOUT THE AUTHOR

Alexandra Yu is a registered nurse with many years of experience in the clinical research industry. Her passion for holistic health led her to launch the Her Holistic Healing podcast. Alexandra's mission is to encourage women to seek God's wisdom *first* for their health and life so that they can experience true, lasting healing that will allow them to make a greater eternal impact in their homes and communities.

Alexandra is a wife and mom of three children. She loves to read, work out, travel, and play the piano, and she has a passion for helping at-risk children.

CONNECT WITH THE AUTHOR

Free resources:
www.herholistichealing.com/freebie

Podcast (all major podcast platforms):
Her Holistic Healing

Website:
www.herholistichealing.com